I0426357

Live Well;

Live Happy!

By:

Cathy Duesterhoeft

This book is dedicated to Claire, my oldest granddaughter.
May you always be happy! Grandma loves you.

Introduction

During a recent sleepover at grandma's house my oldest granddaughter made me aware of her happiness as well as my own. She had just awoken from her nap and she sat in her crib talking and laughing to herself while I listened outside the door. She was in such a good mood, and as a result, so was I. I decided right there and then that when I grow up, I want to be just like Claire; Happy! But then I got to thinking, why shouldn't she be happy. She was only two years old; she had nothing to be sad about. She was at grandma's house, she knows she is well loved and besides, grandma gives her lots of snacks. Still, it made me pause and think about my happiness and how I achieve it. I decided to explore happiness and see if I could figure out what makes people happy. Join me on my journey.

Why Happiness?

True joy and happiness are valuable. To be happy is relatively easy; just decide to be a happy person. Abraham Lincoln observed that most people for most of the time can choose how happy or stressed, how relaxed or troubled, how bright or dull their outlook to be. The choice is simple really, choose to be happy.

Happiness in life is one of the most important things people seek, or should be seeking. True Happiness is hard to achieve and some people search their entire life and never find it. But there are people that do find true happiness in their lives. Some of these people find it without any money or great success. Actually, some people find happiness in life while they are homeless, broke, and alone.

Happiness is part of human nature – people from every background, even from the opposite ends of the Earth, are equally well acquainted with how it feels and are able to recognize it in each other. Happiness in life is easy to experience but almost impossible to hold onto and keep. Everyone (even yourself) has been happy for a moment or two. The secret is being able to recognize happiness in your life and holding onto that feeling and not making yourself miserable.

Happiness is an emotion, but it is greatly influenced by the choices you make. You can choose to be optimistic rather than pessimistic, hopeful rather than doubtful. Sure, life will throw you some curve balls, but no one can steal your happiness.

Remember, it's the journey that should bring you happiness, not the destination. Thinking that when I get a better job, get healthier, find the right person, etc. then I'll be happy is cutting yourself short. What if this takes you 10 years? Will you want to wait that long to feel these wonderful feelings of happiness? No of course not, quit kidding yourself if you said yes. It's about having happy moments as much as you possibly can. Don't wait for some big happy moment to set you off. Be happy just to be alive and able to read this. So many people overlook the meaning of their life and they get stuck in their daily grind to get to the next paycheck, then to the next vacation. If that's you, stop thinking that way, quit reading this and go out for a walk. Enjoy the day even if it's cold.

Another technique to having happiness in life is to surround yourself with happy people and things. If you surround yourself with lots of drama and negativity you won't be able to realize your full happiness potential. Happiness in life isn't going to come on its own. In most cases you will have to work towards it.

A newspaper in England once asked this question of its readers, "Who are the happiest people on the earth?" The four prize-winning answers were:

☺ A little child building sand castles
☺ A craftsman or artist whistling over a job well done
☺ A mother, bathing her baby after a busy day
☺ A doctor who has finished a difficult and dangerous operation that saved a human life

The paper's editors were surprised to find virtually no one submitted kings, emperors, millionaires, or others of riches and rank as the happiest people on earth.

W. Beran Wolfe once said, "If you observe a really happy man you will find him building a boat, writing a symphony, educating his son, growing double dahlias in his garden, or looking for dinosaur eggs in the Gobi desert. He will not be searching for happiness as if it were a collar button that has rolled under a radiator. He will not be striving for it as a goal in itself. He will have become aware that he is happy in the course of living life 24 crowded hours of the day."

Be so happy that when others look at you they become happy too.

Defining Happiness

According to the dictionary, Happiness means the following:

1. the quality or state of being happy.

2. good fortune; pleasure; contentment; joy.

Happiness is thought of as the good life, freedom from suffering, flourishing, well-being, joy, prospective, and pleasure.

Its pursuit is enshrined as a fundamental right in the United States and occupies most of us. But what do we really know about happiness? Can we study it? Are we born with it? Can we make ourselves happier? Who's happy and who's not, and why? What makes us happy? Researchers are learning more and more about the answers to these questions.

Psychologists say yes, and that there are good reasons for doing so. Positive psychology is "the scientific study of the strengths and virtues that enable individuals and communities to thrive." These researchers' work includes studying strengths, positive emotions, resilience, and happiness. Their argument is that only studying psychological disorders gives us just part of the picture of mental health. We will learn more about well-being by studying our strengths and what makes us happy. The hope is that by better understanding human strengths, we can learn new ways to recover from or prevent disorders, and may even learn to become happier.

Researchers also distinguish between the moment-by-moment feeling of happiness produced by positive emotions and how we describe our lives when we think about it. Regardless of whether you had a good day or not, do you describe your life as a happy one? Or describe yourself as a happy person?

Since happiness is so subjective, can it really be measured and studied scientifically? Researchers say yes. They believe that we can reliably and honestly self-report our state of happiness and increases and decreases in happiness. After all, isn't our own perception of happiness what matters? And if we can report it, scientists can measure it.

The Generational Debate

Ask your parents or grandparents to define happiness and they'll surely talk about love, friends, and family. Next, they'll probably mention succeeding in their chosen career, owning a nice home, and having a solid nest egg.

But ask a Gen Y, and the definition of success and happiness may sound quite different. As journalist Hannah Seligson recently wrote of her peers in the Washingtonian, "Instead of a steady job, they want a meaningful one that serves a larger purpose or fulfills a personal passion. And instead of settling down with a spouse and mortgage, they want more years of freedom to chase career dreams and explore different paths before they have to make tradeoffs."

For Millennials, things like climbing the corporate ladder, socking away money for a home, and building up retirement savings have one serious drawback: they take a lot of time. And, experience shows, Millennials don't like to wait. Perhaps because so many of their parents showered them in self-esteem, or perhaps because they witnessed the horrors of 9/11 at a young age and learned that life can be too short, Millennials tend to have a carpe diem philosophy. They want it all, and they want it now.

Some of these generational differences can be seen in the following pages when students of varying ages and adults were asked to define happiness. The youngest of the children found happiness in material things but the teenagers stated they found happiness in family and friends.

According to Students...

Happiness is...

...school
Tyler-age 5

...reading books
Emalie-age 5

...playing with my cousin's bunny
Cristen-age 6

...playing with my cousin
Jazmin-age 6

...getting my new BB gun
Ashton-age 7

...playing soccer
Taylor-age 7

...video games
Will-age 7

...playing with my brother
Ella-age 7

...video games
Chaderick-age 7

...candy
Brandon-age 7

…going to a water park
Hayli-age 7

…seeing my dad
Travis-age 8

…playing video games
Shane-age 9

…sports and fun activities
Angie-age 9

…ponies, unicorns, rainbows, balloons, candy, ice cream and
going to water parks
Courtney-age 9

…play football and playing outside
Jasper-age 9

…when I get my new toys
Johnathan-age 9

…when I wrestle with my brother
Carter-age 10

…when I have fun
Madelyn-age 10

…playing outside with my cats and friends
Harley-age 10

...being myself and doing what I want to do
Anna-age 10

...playing basketball, being outside, hunting, four wheeling, going to the farm
Katie-age 10

...art, dancing
Rachel-age 10

...hunting and fishing
Cody-age 10

...when I have fun
Austin-age 10

...when I get to play baseball
Tyler-age 10

...I like doing a lot of stuff but I like baseball most
Jesse-age 10

...to play football and to be outdoors and help the environment
Abe-age 10

...my family
Haley-age 10

...free video games and/or world peace and/or curing world hunger
Harrison-age 10

…when I get to see my little sister, mom and dad
Maddie-age 10

…when it is someone's birthday
Deyonna-age 11

…going fishing when in stress
Chase-age 11

…gymnastics, outdoors, hunting, and fishing
Brooke-age 11

…when my mom really loves me and does stuff with me
Dee Dee-age 11

…having fun, smiling, being kind
Claudia-age 11

…my cat
Kenny-age 11

…smiling
Camryn-age 11

…being nice to people
Melissa-age 11

…a feeling that is good to me
Breanna-age 11

…when you are happy to do something
Lacey-age 11

…when no one calls you a mean name
Evelinn-age 11

…staying home gaming all day
Zach-age 11

…being nice
Jesse-age 11

…when something good happens to you
Owen-age 11

…riding a horse
Logan-age 11

…the hilarious times in your little life
Kevin-age 11

…when we are joyful and are not sad or short of the love we all share
Lily-age 11

…when you don't feel bad, when you have a good time, and especially when you have good friends
Evan-age 11

…love from family
Elias-age 11

…when my family is doing good and friends are having fun
Lindsay-age 11

...when you are laughing and having fun
Keaton-age 11

...singing, crumpling paper and playing a game, having fun
Bailey-age 11

...fun, cool
Robynn-age11

...when you get an assignment done, having fun, getting a present
Nick-age 11

...doing things we like
Savanna-age 11

...when someone jokes and laughs when they get hurt
Amanda-age 11

...having fun
Dylan-age 12

...the feeling when friends are laughing and being a team
Catelin-age 12

...the TV show New Jersey
David-age 12

...singing, football, band, great friends
Rayann-age 12

...friendship
Mason-age 12

...a feeling you get when something goes right for you
Megan-age 13

...being part of a team
Brianne-age 13

...caring and making sure people are happy
Ashley-age 14

...making memories that will stay with you forever
Hailey-age 14

...when you are doing something you enjoy, or making other people smile
Timmlyn-age 14

...friends, family, and love!
Joline-age 14

...family, joy
Kira-age 14

...an emotion that no one can fulfill but yourself
Ashley-age 14

...doing something you love day in and day out
Jake-age 14

...being around the people you love and care about
Autumn-age 14

...being loved
Bailey-age 14

...when you have fun in life with no worries
Jason-age 14

...being organized
Bret-age 14

...a feeling of joy and getting a good response to something
Mythel-age 14

...dogs
Dustin-age 14

...no rules, no worries, doing what I want (and money)
Austin-age 14

...being in a place where you feel comfortable and safe with
who you are and what you feel
Emma-age 14

...hanging out with or hanging around stuff you like to do
Alysha-age 14

...when you feel great about yourself
Clarissa-age 14

...getting good grades, getting rewards for things
Kennedy-age 14

...a crappie on the hook
Calvin-age 15

...enjoying life
Dylan-age 15

...being able to be yourself and not be restricted from what
you want to do and who you want to be
Micia-Roy-age 15

...having fun, taking risks while still knowing your
consequences and accepting who you are and who is there
through it all
Jesse-age 15

...being outside
Michael-age 15

...always being happy and having a good time
Annie-age 15

...when I do something good and right
Jonah-age 15

...doing whatever I want
Noah-age 15

...a key to live a great life
Dylan-age 15

...everything sports, having fun
Alan-age 15

...friends
Darren-age 15

...not wanting to spend a day in someone else's skin
Samantha-age 15

...being around people that love and accept you without
judgment, laughing with friends and family, being
comfortable as you
Brittany-age 15

...anything that brings you joy, anything that is exciting and
you enjoy
Caitlin-age 15

...never getting mad, not worrying about everything and
having no stress, being nice to everyone
Bronwyn-age 15

...me being alone and inventing
Devin-age 15

...the key of life, rebel, music
Sara-age 15

...freedom, music, rebelling, no rules
Leah-age 15

...roller coasters
Steven-age 15

...fun, doing what you like
Devin-age 15

...people who are honest (and cupcakes)
Aryanna-age 15

...being alone and being independent-age 15
Jenny-age 15

...friends, family, life and love
Dillon-age 15

...food
Johnny-age 15

...being with your family and not letting others influence you,
be a leader
Nate-age 15

...my friends and family
Kristina-age 15

...to be loved by friends, family and to do things I enjoy
Aiden-age 15

...the other side of the rainbow and no rules
Adam-age 15

…doing what you want and not letting anyone tell you otherwise
Matt-age 15

…when I can play video games by myself in my room
Brone-age 15

…sports, hanging out with friends, gaming, being in control
David-age 16

…not caring
Danny-age 16

…the enjoyment of life and what it brings
Lauren-age 15

…something that makes me smile, like when everyone is in a good mood and laugh about things
Dahna-age 15

…feeling loved by others, to do things that you enjoy and to feel like you matter
Brittany-age 16

…feeling at peace and comfortable and not having to worry about big problems
Amber-age 16

…a good life, well lived
Caitlin-age 16

...having all your needs filled. When you don't need anything else, you're happy
Carolyn-age 16

...seeing all my friends and family happy which makes me happy
Jazmon-age 16

...not having fear, failure to ever appear real.
Anna-age 16

...feeling the love of someone else and helping them in any way you can
Ashley-age 16

...disregarding the problems you are going through and enjoying life
Domonique-age 16

...helping others from an honest heart and going after what you are truly interested in
Ania-age 16

...the satisfaction of making an impact in someone else's life and to love unconditionally
Crystal-age 17

...when someone says they love you and you feel it. Also, when you don't feel the need to impress...just be.
Connor-age 17

...the feeling in your true heart and soul that you are in a state of true bliss
John-age 17

...acceptance and the safety it brings when you can relax and just smile and laugh
Kelly-age 17

...what I'm going to feel when snow finally falls and I'll be able to snowmobile
Chase-age 17

...loving life, following your dreams or doing what you love even if you don't have wealth, fame and fortune
Amber-age 17

...knowing someone loves you and knowing you have the ability to affect change. Basically when you look at life and think, it's all good
Dawn-age 17

...the one peace you can always confide in and my peace
Crystal-age 18

...having a satisfying relationship with God that makes you feel safe and loved and having that reaffirmed by people around you, and reaffirming that in others
Alyssa-age 18

...the feeling that you get when nothing can bring you down
Austin-age 18

…finding love in yourself and those around you
Morgan-age 19

…being with the people you care about and knowing that no matter what they will be there for you and love you no matter what and it's the little things in life that make you smile and laugh no matter what
Samantha-age 20

…a family together sharing life, loving each other
Steven-age 20

…Being around people who you love and who love you
Mallory-age 21

…finding love and caring for you loved ones as well as being loved
Ashley-age 23

…relaxing with my family
Nathan-age 26

…the love and acceptance of yourself only when we love and accept ourselves can we open to love and accept other.
Hazel-age 38

I decided to seek further information from a handful of adults so I asked more questions. A list of their answers is below:

1. How do you define happiness?

*A state of mind and a way of life
*Being happy
*The health of my kids and husband
*Kids
*A warm feeling of being content
*Smiles; wellbeing
*A feeling I get when I have my family is around me
*Being content and at peace with yourself and all of the external things that play a role in your life such as, relationships, jobs, family, etc.
*Peace within
*A sense of well-being, feeling good about life in general, getting joy from basic stuff (the green grass, the blue of the sky, etc.)
*When I feel contented or at ease, or when I feel needed and/or serving a useful purpose to others, or when all is right in my little world
*I define happiness basically as contentedness. When you can just "be" and not be waiting for the "next thing" that will change your life and finally make everything okay. I also define happiness as the ability to see joy in the things around you, no matter how minimal they seem to the outside world.
*Being yourself and no one tries to change you
*Being grateful for what I have
*Spending time with family and friends and enjoying life in general.
*A positive state of mind
*It is accepting and appreciating the good in life and truly believing that if God brought you to it--he'll get you through it and even though you don't always understand why life may be dealing you a raw deal--someone else has it worse.
*A state of bliss like love hard to describe but you know it

because it feels right.

*I make distinction between happiness and joy. Happiness I assign to the mind; joy I assign to the spirit (accepting the classic Greek formula that a human being is of mind, body and spirit). Happiness is temporary; joy is eternal. Happiness pertains to self; joy pertains to relationship with others. When someone is happy, events or circumstances has affirmed the desires and goals of the individual. I'm happy when the lawnmower starts on the first pull. I'm joyful to see my children achieve a goal, such as graduation from high school. So I would define happiness as affirmation of self.

*Happiness is being contented with life, as it is. Not yearning for something else. *For me, in particular, I am happiest when I feel like a competent person.

2. Do you believe that like diet and exercise, happiness is a way of life or is it situational?

*It's a way of life: a choice

*It's situational

*Way of life

*Situational

*It's a choice and how you look at life

*A bit of both

*Happiness should be a way of life but it isn't always

*It can be both a way of life and be situational. I think for some people they get happiness from the events that happen in their life and I believe that for some people they just have an optimistic outlook on everything and are in general happy with everything.

*There are two kinds of happiness, one as a way of life and one situational. I can be happy in my soul, yet when things go wrong there is a sadness as well.

*I feel very strongly that it is a way of life and sometimes it is something we have to work at

*I think it can be both. If I had to choose, I would consider happiness more a way of life. I would describe "situational" happiness more as a feeling of excitement, pride, etc.

*I believe happiness is a way of life that can be enhanced situationally. Overall, I think people are either happy or unhappy at their core and that unhappy people are generally unhappy even when "happy" things happen to them-they just see the negative in it and refuse to see the positive in anything. One the flip side, happy people will find happiness even when the situation they are in is rough. It's deeper than what is going on in your life on a day-to-day basis. That being said, I think that happiness can be influenced situationally for most people, although that is usually a temporary flux and doesn't really change a person's core happiness level.

*I believe it is situational

*It is a state of mind. I guess that would make it a way of life.

*Happiness is a way of life.

*Way of life

*No, happiness comes from within--it's how you handle your own state of being.

*Know it is situational, there are different states/levels of happiness

*I believe it is both. A person who places unachievable thresholds on self-affirmation has established a "way of life" and will never be happy. It's tough for a person who is insecure to be happy. Security alone will not cause happiness.

*However, with personal security established, situations can, and will cause happiness.

*There are certainly people who exude happiness; for them it is a way of life. For most, happiness does increase or decrease according to the situation.

3. If you think happiness is situational, what types of things make you happy?
*Anything can make you happy; finding the silver lining
*Family, love
*Being covered in sawdust (submitted by a wood crafter)
*My kids and kids in general
*Children and animals
*Family
*Of course family and friends, but also purchasing my own house, my dog, family vacations/trips, listening to certain music, certain events in my life, like my wedding day.
*Being with family, quiet time when I can find it, a good book.
*Lots of things! This could be a certain event. It could be anything from a single event like finding a dime on the ground (instead of a penny); to my daughter getting an unexpected "A" on a difficult math test.
*While I don't think situations really determine someone's deepest level of happiness-sort of their resting point in terms of their happiness level-I think certain situations can affect it at least temporarily. Very serious things like how a person feels they are being treated either in personal or professional relationships can influence you one way or another and bring you up or down. If you are dealing with a deeply painful thing like a death or illness of someone close to you, even a person who tends to be happy can be brought down-although I believe the happy person will weather it better and come out of the "down" sooner. I don't think that stuff like getting stuck in traffic or finding $10 on the sidewalk has a real impact on a person's meaningful happiness level.
*What makes me happy is seeing my grandchildren and when my kids are happy in their lives.
*Watching my grandchildren play, my wife after a fresh haircut, the accomplishment of a new challenge.

*Um…when the lawnmower starts on the first pull…when a thought-out plan comes to fruition…when the sun shines on a day that I've chosen for an outside activity (like golf or camping).

*Being outdoors (gardening, being on the lake, hiking); feeling that I have accomplished something worthwhile.

4. If you are going through a down or sad period, how do you "get your happy on?"

*Think about what is good in life; I take time for myself and think

*Being with my family

*Think about something funny that my kids have done or said

*Shoot guns (submitted by a hunter)

*Smile. My daughter told me once that I make her smile and that makes her happy.

*Friends, family, music

*I try to surround myself with family and close friends. Sometimes shopping makes me happy and feel good! Sometimes just being alone and thinking things out.

*Pray

*Exercise, time alone to reflect (but not too much time alone), helping others, appreciating nature and the wonders of our world, spending time with family, staying busy

*Try to put things in perspective by thinking about how the problem causing the down/sad period will affect my life a year from now. What are the chances I will even remember it. If so, think about how much worse the situation could have been, then look on the bright side. Then try to look at all of the other positives in my life and try to move on. Take a deep breath and blow out all the misery!

*For me, fresh air, movement, and spending time with nature is helpful. A hike somewhere beautiful is the best medicine for me. Basically, disconnecting from life stressors and allowing my mind to be quiet and clear itself while my body moves and breathes. Just getting even mild exercise can get me through a lot. Also, working through whatever is getting me down by talking with my husband is really helpful. I also like to recharge by quietly reading or by switching up the norm in my routine and doing anything that is novel or fresh that I

haven't had a chance to do in a while.

*Having my grandchildren around

*Read the scriptures, say my prayers and go for a walk.

*Think about what life has done for me and how lucky I am to be alive and generally healthy.

*Being with supportive friends, doing anything!

*Pray that the good Lord helps me to accept the things I cannot change, change the things I can and the wisdom to know the difference.

*Time, and then I move on

*Change my environment and/or activity. Call a friend. Build or fix something in my shop.

*I don't really have down times, but in times of stress, reading escapist fiction or getting outdoors are good.

5. Are you usually a happy person?

*Yes

*I like to think so

*Yupper

*Yes

*Usually always

*Yes, most often

*Yes

*I have to admit that I actually am very pessimistic at times and when going through things but then I have many times that I can look at the positive side of situations and think, that's why that happened.

*Yes

*Yes

*Yes, I feel like I am. I find that I generally tend to talk about the crazy negatives that might happen in the day-to-day goings on of my life. But I believe that this is my way of purging the bad and clearing the plate.

*I would say that I am a happy person. I try to see joy in the little things and usually succeed in that. I try not to let life's inconveniences like an unexpected car repair or a change in plans get me down. I think each day is a gift-I am thankful to be here and glad I get to live this life and I don't ever find myself wishing for a different version of my life. I would say I am content and blessed.

*Most of the time I am happy

*Yes

*Yes

*Yes, I don't think I can say that I have ever been depressed.

*I think so

*Yes

*I typically seek the lighter side of life and usually find it. Yes, I'm happy.

6. Please share a story about something that made you happy. *My daughter playing makes me happy. Seeing her smile and laugh and having a good time.

*Any moment with family.

*My husband proposing and the birth of each of my kids.

*When my patient walked when the odds were against her.

*The birth of my 3 children.

*The trip that we made to Italy was the greatest. Our son-in-law and daughter planned the trip. It was where my dad grew up. He came to the states when he was 18 years old. It was amazing how we were treated. We loved it!

*My wedding was something that made me happy. Everything about the day, everyone that joined us to celebrate our day, all of our family and close friends were there with us, the dancing and one thing that was very special to me on that day was a special dance with my brother. He was a very influential male figure in my life and it meant a lot to have those few minutes to have a special time with him and that made me very happy.

*Just recently, my husband and I celebrated our 29th anniversary. To celebrate, we spent the whole day together and at his suggestion, bought me a whole new wardrobe. The clothes are NOT what made me happy. I have been uncomfortable with my appearance for a long time and not able to do anything about it for some reason. He has told me all along, that it does not matter to him what I look like--he loves me anyway, and part of the reason my weight is an issue is because of the 6 wonderful children I have given him. The clothes were a tangible form of that love--he wants me to feel as good as I look to him, no matter what I weigh. It was completely unexpected and he usually hates to shop. No one would have known that though, he walked throughout the store bringing me more and more things to try on. It was a very happy day and just thinking about the boost he gave to my ego is enough to keep me smiling no matter what.

*When I am driving behind a school bus that is making stops dropping off children at their homes. I love watching the little ones as they walk up the driveway, dragging their backpacks, stopping to look at bugs, and just being children.

*Went to the mall today at lunch (3-days before Christmas) and made it in and out quickly by going the back way. So happy not to have to wait in that long line at the front of the mall.

*My family likes to hike around Ennis Lake at John Muir Park several times a year. All my kids have hiked around it on foot (I think it's almost 3 miles) before they could talk. It always makes me proud that I grow such hearty kids who love to be physically active and are tough little buggers who don't whine to be carried. We take the dog, the kids, and go out there and take our time, listen to our voices echo, check out the water, look for creatures of all kinds, etc. My kids are so happy out there and I love watching them run freely and enjoy themselves and each other. Always love watching the baby chase the bigger ones. Always feel like God is smiling on me. It always reminds me what is important and sends me the message to simplify and enjoy my kids and my life. I do not need to be plugged into technology or have a ton of stuff to be happy. I need my family and our time together.

*When we have a picnic and my family comes over that is something that makes me happy. We have a picnic maybe once a month.

*My husband and my family are what make me most happy.

*We are in the process of building our retirement home. It makes me happy to think that someday we will have a place to go to and enjoy the rest of our lives together up north and in the woods.

*Several years ago, my mother was critically ill and after being with her in the hospital, much of the night, there was a breakfast of friends scheduled at 7:00 a.m. There was no question that I would go, it lifted my spirits, supported me, made me laugh. Luckily for me, these friends are always around, we laugh and play and cry together.

*The love of my family makes me happy. When you think that you can't love anyone or anything more than your spouse and your children, along comes children-in-law and grandchildren and to love them and be loved by them is totally overwhelming. My oldest grandson carried the Christ candle in church and to see how proud he was to do it brought tears to my eyes because not only was he proud to carry the candle, he knew how proud we were of him. *Happiness is also spending time with your children-in-law families and finding that you love them as much or more than your own siblings and knowing that your WHOLE family has a totally special meaning because now a days families aren't as connected. I love that my children react to their sibling's extended families as if they were their own.

*As I enjoy my new level of fitness I have been extremely happy that my wife has started to take my feelings and desires into consideration.

*The lawnmower started on the first pull! No, I guess that's part of seeking the lighter side of the conversation. Last summer I graduated from the United Methodist Course of Study for Licensed Local Pastors (happy, happy!) This summer I'm reading fiction for personal enjoyment!

*It is alarming to me that I can't readily think of anything that isn't a cliché. I will say that my happiest times have been outdoors.

Laughter, the Best Medicine

A healthy dose of humor can make a significant contribution to your overall health and well-being. Science is learning what common sense has shown us all along; Laughter is wonderful medicine and an important aid to healing. It revitalizes and relieves tension. No matter what problems you face today, look for humor.

It's all in the Attitude

Set a tone of happiness for the day by smiling as soon as you wake up each morning. First, smile at God, saying in your heart, *Thank You for watching over me all night.* Second, smile at the remembrance of at least one good thing that happened the day before. Third, smile at the thought of all the opportunities and blessings that await you during the day. Fourth, smile at the thought that God will be present throughout the day to help you with every crisis, challenge, or obstacle. Fifth, smile at the very fact that you are alive and *smiling.*

And since you will have so many smiles, be sure and give some away!

The Power of Relationships

Finding happiness in a relationship may seem pointless when that relationship is unhealthy. On the other hand there is a way to make changes within yourself, that may help. Finding happiness in your relationship is easy if you are happy within yourself to begin with. What if you're not happy with yourself? How do you work on self-fulfillment while trying to fix a broken relationship? Isn't that selfish?

Think of your relationship as a recipe. When you mix healthy ingredients together, the result is a healthy and tasty dish. When one or both of the ingredients is spoiled, your culinary creation is spoiled as well. Likewise, a healthy relationship is created when both people are mentally healthy. By nurturing yourself, you are improving your relationship recipe. Therefore, self-improvement is not a selfish act, but one that strengthens your relationship as a whole.

Happiness in your relationship is a two way street. While you are working on your own self help, don't forget about your partner. If they lack self-esteem, take the time to reassure them of their self-worth. Let them know that you appreciate the things they do for you. Take the time to make them feel good about themselves. It's vital to know you are valued in a relationship. Even if you have been together a long time, it helps to verify your importance to each other occasionally.

Sometimes we get caught up in everyday life and forget about ourselves for a while. The bills must be paid. The chores must be done. We must make sure all is right with family and friends. When this happens, our own happiness and sense of self-worth sometimes fall by the wayside. What have you done for yourself lately? When you feel neglected due to the stress of everyday living, it's hard to find happiness in your relationship. Take the time to nurture yourself and your relationship will profit from your inner happiness.

Find out what foods can boost your mood and help fight depression.

One in twenty Americans suffers from depression. If you're feeling blue—or want to ward off feeling that way—there are some foods to consider that might help. Studies have linked the foods on the following slides with helping people cope with the blues. Here are some to try. (As with any health condition, you should, of course, consult your healthcare provider for a full treatment plan.)

1. Coffee

A recent study which appeared in the Archives of Internal Medicine suggested that women who drink coffee have lower rates of depression. Sure, it was an association, which doesn't prove that coffee was responsible for the lower rates of depression, but it was a very large study (more than 50,000 women) that traced coffee intake and depression diagnoses over the course of 14 years. That is strong enough evidence to say that if you already drink coffee, you can count this among the other potential health boons to support your coffee habit.

2. Salmon

Omega-3 fatty acids help our brain cells communicate and enhance the concentration of dopamine and serotonin—two neurotransmitters that help regulate mood. Seafood, such as salmon and sardines, is high in omega-3s, as are walnuts and ground flaxseed. In one study, researchers found that participants who had lower blood levels of omega-3 fatty acids were more likely to report mild or moderate symptoms of depression.

3. Saffron

Saffron, those expensive red threads that lend Persian cooking an intense golden color, may not be a spice you cook with often. But using it could raise your spirits. As Joyce Hendley reported in Eating Well Magazine, saffron has long been used in traditional Persian medicine as a mood lifter, usually steeped into a medicinal tea or used to prepare rice. Tehran University of Medical Sciences researcher Shahin Akhondzadeh, Ph.D., has found that saffron has antidepressant effects comparable to the antidepressants fluoxetine (Prozac) and imipramine (Tofranil), likely because it makes the feel-good neurotransmitter serotonin more available to the brain (the same mechanism that makes Prozac work).

4. Carbs

Cutting out carbs can have an unintended consequence: a foul mood. Researchers suspect that is because carbs promote the production of serotonin. In a study from the Archives of

Internal Medicine, people who followed a very low-carbohydrate diet for a year—which allowed only 20 to 40 grams of carbs daily, about the amount in just 1/2 cup of rice plus one slice of bread—experienced more depression, anxiety and anger than those assigned to a low-fat, high-carb diet that focused on low-fat dairy, whole grains, fruit and beans.

5. Chocolate

Chocolate certainly brings a smile to many faces. And there's actually a scientific reason why! Chocolate's antioxidants may help lower levels of cortisol—the so-called stress hormone. Stressed-out people who ate 1.4 ounces of dark chocolate daily for two weeks had lower levels of stress hormones, including cortisol, in a study done recently at the Nestlé Research Center in Switzerland. Choose dark chocolate with the highest cacao content to get the most antioxidant—and be mindful of the 230 calories in 1.4 ounces of chocolate.

Don't Forget About Fido

Whether finned, feathered or furry, pets are good for your health. People who own pets have healthier hearts and make fewer visits to the doctor. During times of stress, a pet can lower blood pressure. Pet owners are more physically fit and tend to be less lonely or fearful than those without pets. And if you want to get in shape, dogs make better exercise partners than humans-they never want to skip a walk. "Animals provide us with much of the same kind of social support that people do, "says Alan Beck, director of Purdue University's Center for the Human-Animal Bond. And they're always there when you need them.

Happy Now Sad Later
(Situational)

IS THE GLASS HALF FULL OR HALF EMPTY?

This is the classic question that determines whether one is an optimist or pessimist.

The purpose of the question is to demonstrate that the situation may be seen in different ways depending on one's point of view and that there may be opportunity in the situation as well as trouble. This idiom is used to explain how people perceive events and objects. Perception is unique to every individual and is simply one's interpretation of reality.

Situational happiness is when we depend on external circumstances in order to provide us with joy and well-being. We crave our "external world" to be a certain way, and if we don't get it then we are left disappointed and unhappy. Those who learn to cultivate emotional independence (especially dedicated meditation practitioners like Buddhist monks), find out how to find happiness that is independent of these external conditions.

Some of the most common things we become dependent on for happiness include:

- Excessive eating.

- Alcohol and drugs.

- Movies, TV, music, video games, the internet, and other entertainment.

- Sex.

- Shopping and consumerism.

- People.

- Pets.

- Wealth and money.

- Traditions and routine.

- Etc.

These are all desires that we can develop a near-addictive personality toward. Of course, someone can develop an addictive personality toward nearly anything, but of course that doesn't make any of these habits *necessarily* bad. Only when can no longer exercise these habits in moderation, and we begin to depend on them to enjoy ourselves, do these habits turn into a problem. Then, we are emotionally dependent on them in order to live a fulfilling life.

The idea that one's emotional state should be determined by events is pervasive; it's no coincidence that the words happen and happy share a common root. Almost every action life performs is designed to improve its external conditions: every amoeba wriggling up a chemical gradient, every car on the road driven by someone to somewhere they'd rather be.

But letting today's events determine today's mood is problematic because circumstances are transient and so the happiness dissolves when the circumstances change, as they inevitably do. Seeking refuge in the impermanent and the unreliable lets minute-by-minute events hijack your emotions, your mind, yourself. To the extent that your emotions drive your behavior, situational happiness reduces your authenticity, by expressing a conditional, contingent version of you, not the absolute, essential you.

Habitually happy people know how they like to feel. They like to feel good and on top of their game all of the time. They like to be and try to be energized, up, happy and enthusiastic all of the time. They continually try to do their best, feel their best and be at their best. Try to become a habitually happy person in order to avoid situational happiness.

Spiritual Happiness

There have been countless research studies on spiritual well-being or just being happy, and all have shown that feeling good about yourself or everyday situations maintains or improves one's health. Everyone seems to have a different way of finding happiness. Some people find it in religion while others might find it in food, exercise, favorite hobbies, family, and friends.

A spiritually happy person is in tune with and accepting of themselves. They feel no need to impress anyone or to compete. They love themselves (not in an egotistical way) the way they are.

With spiritual happiness, you are not waiting to be rich before you can be happy, or to find the right person to be happy, or to have more friends to be happy. You don't need to look different to be spiritually happy; nor do you have to heal all your flaws to be spiritually happy. With spiritual happiness, you can look at the world with realistic eyes -- seeing, experiencing, and responding to all the muddled mess that life can sometimes seem to be. Yet, in the depths of your being, you'll know a peacefulness and contentment that never fades, even while the world may be crashing down around you.

Bible Verses Pertaining to Happiness

Behold, God will not cast away a perfect [man], neither will
he help the evil doers: Till he fill thy mouth with laughing,
and thy lips with rejoicing.
Job 8:20-21

Make me to hear joy and gladness; [that] the bones [which] thou
hast broken may rejoice.
Psalms 51:8

Make a joyful noise unto the Lord, all the earth: make a loud
noise, and rejoice, and sing praise. Sing unto the Lord with
the harp; with the harp, and the voice of a psalm. With trumpets
and sound of cornet make a joyful noise before the Lord,
the King. Let the sea roar, and the fullness thereof; the world,
and they that dwell therein. Let the floods clap [their] hands:
let the hills be joyful together
Psalms 98:4-8

A Psalm of praise. Make a joyful noise unto the Lord, all ye lands.
Serve the Lord with gladness: come before his presence with singing.
Psalms 100:1-2

The hope of the righteous [shall be] gladness: but the expectation of
the wicked shall perish.
Proverbs 10:28

A merry heart maketh a cheerful countenance: but by sorrow of the heart the spirit is broken.
Proverbs 15:13

All the days of the afflicted [are] evil: but he that is of a merry heart [hath] a continual feast.
Proverbs 15:15

A merry heart doeth good [like] a medicine: but a broken spirit drieth the bones.
Proverbs 17:22

In the day of prosperity be joyful, but in the day of adversity consider: God also hath set the one over against the other, to the end that man should find nothing after him.
Ecclesiastes 7:14

Therefore with joy shall ye draw water out of the wells of salvation.
Isaiah 12:3

Blessed are ye, when men shall hate you, and when they shall separate you [from their company], and shall reproach [you], and cast out your name as evil, for the Son of man's sake. Rejoice ye in that day, and leap for joy: for, behold, your reward [is] great in heaven: for in the like manner did their fathers unto the prophets.
Luke 6:22-23

If ye keep my commandments, ye shall abide in my love; even as I have kept my Father's commandments, and abide in his love. These things have I spoken unto you, that my joy might remain in you, and [that] your joy might be full.
John 15:10-11

And ye now therefore have sorrow: but I will see you again, and your heart shall rejoice, and your joy no man taketh from you.
John 16:22

These things I have spoken unto you, that in me ye might have peace. In the world ye shall have tribulation: but be of good cheer; I have overcome the world.
John 16:33

Rejoice with them that do rejoice, and weep with them that weep.
Romans 12:15

Rejoice in the Lord always: [and] again I say, Rejoice.
Philippians 4:4

Strengthened with all might, according to his glorious power, unto all patience and longsuffering with joyfulness;
Colossians 1:11

Rejoice evermore.
1 Thessalonians 5:16

Can Money Buy Happiness?

Much research has found that richer people tend to be happier.

Happiness now equals more money later: If you want your kids to grow up to be rich, make sure he/she is happy now. A study that analyzed data from 15,000 kids, and followed up with them ten years later, found that those rated highest on scales of emotional well-being and life satisfaction were more likely to earn higher incomes as adults. One theory on the connection is that happy people may be more likely than unhappy ones to pursue higher education and also more likely, once in the workforce, to get the promotions needed to bring in the big bucks.

The ingredients necessary to produce genuine happiness vary from person to person, but one thing is true for all-material wealth or possessions never fully satisfy the inner longings of the human heart. Neither do they establish self-worth or fulfill our inner need for love.

You may not be able to buy happiness but that doesn't stop companies from trying to sell it to you. Check out the list of companies and the happiness tag line they use.

Arby's-It's Good Mood Food
Crete Carrier-The key to happiness is in this ignition
Golden Corral-Help yourself to happiness

Coke-Open happiness
Frito-Lay-Happiness is simple
Campbell's Soup-Putting you on the road to happiness
Prevacid-Happiness is a day without heartburn
US Cellular-Be with the happiest customer
Febreeze-Breathe happy
Brooks-Run happy
Walgreen's-At the corner of Healthy and Happy
Folgers-Wake up with happiness in a cup
ING Direct-…right back on the road to happiness
Zappos-Delivering happiness

I don't know about you, but I know I will not run happy even if I don a pair of Brooks shoes.

One of the Buddhist teachings is that wealth does not guarantee happiness and also wealth is impermanent. The people of every country suffer whether rich or poor, but those who understand Buddhist teachings can find true happiness.

Different How?

Pleasure or Happiness?

We are a pleasure seeking society. Most of us spend our energy seeking pleasure and avoiding pain. We hope that by doing this, we will feel happy. Yet happiness and joy seems to elude many people.

The reason for this is because there is a huge difference between happiness and pleasure. Pleasure is a momentary feeling that comes from something external – a good meal, our stock going up, making love, and so on.

Pleasure has to do with the positive experiences of our senses, and with good things happening. Pleasurable experiences can give us momentary feelings of happiness, but this happiness does not last long because it is dependent upon external events and experiences.

We have to keep on having the good experiences – more food, more drugs or alcohol, more money, more sex, more things – in order to feel pleasure. As a result, many people become addicted to these external experiences, needing more and more to feel a short-lived feeling of happiness.

Happiness, on the other hand is a state of mind. It is a reflection of what is going on inside ourselves. Many people go out to the bar or get together with this person or that person all in attempt to find happiness.

The sad thing is that these people will never find it. That is as long as they keep looking outside of themselves.

Content or Happy?

The American Heritage Dictionary records the definition of the word content as "satisfied" whereas happiness (a derivative of the word happy) means:
1. Characterized by good fortune
2. Having, showing or marked by pleasure

From the above definitions, it appears that happiness is a state of mind or attitude that is induced by the presence of favorable circumstances. To be content (based upon the definition of satisfy) means "to gratify or fulfill a need or desire". Hence, it represents a state of mind that is induced when a need or desire is fulfilled…not necessarily as a result of favorable circumstances.

To be happy denotes a state of being that relies on positive experiences to reinforce its existence. Hence, when difficult times occur, you can fall from the state of happiness into the state of fear (anger, depression and chaos) until the negative stimulus is eliminated. However, to be content denotes a state of mind that is not based upon positive or negative stimulation …it is a feeling akin to peace of mind. To be content means that one accepts all circumstances as part of the natural rhythm of life…the cosmic flow that contains both peaks and valleys.

Joy vs. Happy-

Both joy and happiness are positive and desirable emotions where a person has a feeling of being satisfied. These feelings are based on certain reasons, and the nature that causes that particular feeling can differ.

Joy comes from the inner-self of a person, and is connecting with the source of life within you. It is caused by something really exceptional and satisfying. The source of joy is something or someone greatly appreciated or valued, and it is not only about oneself, but also about the contentment of those people whom you value the most.

Happiness is an emotion experienced when in a state of well-being. The state of well-being is characterized by emotions ranging from contentment to intense joy. Happiness is simply the state of being happy. It may be caused by good fortune, luck or various other pleasures that range from person to person. Happiness is a result of something that is outside of you, and gained by observing or doing that particular thing. Social networks and human relationships are the most important correlation with happiness. Happiness spreads through relationships like friends, siblings, partners, neighbors etc.

Happiness may be momentary, as it is a result of short-term contentment; but joy, being related to the inner self, is long lasting. Happiness simply pleases a person, while joy brings warmth to that person's heart, and brings contentment to one's heart.

Happiness comes from outside, while joy from within, and with this attitude of joy, the person is in a state of grace. Joy is an extension to happiness. It is a continuous state of happiness, and a positive emotion. It is not merely a fleeting thing, like happiness.

31 Types of Happiness-You decide the difference between them.

Anticipation, playful, optimistic, love, humor, helpful, relieved, kindness, giving, hopeful, satisfaction, content, blessed, confident, nostalgic, celebrate, honorable, balanced, motivated, amused, enthusiasm, thankful, awestruck, social, joyful, peaceful, cheerful, lively, spiritual, inspired, mellow.

50 Ideas That Could Bring Happiness
(in no particular order)

☺ Go for a run
☺ Call a friend
☺ Hug someone special
☺ Visit a shut in
☺ Listen to music
☺ Read a good book
☺ Spend time with your grandchildren
☺ Play a card game
☺ Garden
☺ Go shopping
☺ Spend time in nature
☺ Go for a drive
☺ Go to a movie
☺ Buy yourself flowers
☺ Treat yourself to an ice cream cone
☺ Go for a bike ride
☺ Soak in a bubble bath
☺ Sip a glass of wine
☺ Spend time with your spouse
☺ Dance
☺ Cook something healthy
☺ Go to church
☺ Sing
☺ Tell a joke
☺ Bite into a crunchy apple
☺ Have a pedicure
☺ Enjoy sex
☺ Brew a fresh cup of coffee
☺ Get a new hairstyle
☺ Bake a batch of cookies and share them
☺ Light a scented candle
☺ Golf
☺ Treat yourself to a spa day

☺ Play twister with your spouse

☺ Connect with your kids

☺ Visit the zoo and make sure you check out the monkeys!

☺ Pop some popcorn

☺ Go for a walk

☺ Have a manicure

☺ Watch a favorite rerun on TV

☺ Meet a friend for lunch

☺ Go fishing

☺ Volunteer

☺ Try a new hobby

☺ Close your eyes for some quiet me time

☺ Sleep in

☺ Eat at a new restaurant

☺ Hum along to the song on the radio

☺ Pretend you are the "Dancing Baby"

☺ Connect with an old friend on Facebook

Happiness Quotes

"Happiness is like a butterfly; the more you chase it, the more it will elude you, but if you turn your attention to other things, it will come and sit softly on your shoulder."
-Henry David Thoreau

"Happiness comes from within and is found in the present moment by making peace with the past and looking forward to the future."
-Unknown

"Happiness cannot be traveled to, owned, earned, worn or consumed. Happiness is the Spiritual experience of living every minute with love, grace and gratitude.'
-Denis Waitley

"Happiness is not a consequence of things that happen. Do not pursue happiness-practice it. Sing, even if you do not sound good. Smile, even when things go wrong. Create happiness, and happy you will be."
-Unknown

Happy people have higher energy. It is thought that happy people have stronger romantic and social relationships than others and it all stems from a philosophical view of life.
-Unknown

"Success is not the key to happiness. Happiness is the key to success."
-Herman Cain, Newspaper Columnist

Happiness is not a destination in which you arrive. It is your journey there. Whatever benefits you expect to be yours at the end of your journey, simply receive them in the beginning.
-Unknown

Three small rules for living a happy life:
1.) Start each day with a grateful heart.
2.) Focus on the positive aspects of every person you encounter.
3.) End each day with a grateful heart
-Lucy Mac Donald

Little acts of kindness can add up to a lifetime of happiness. "Always leave enough time in your life to do something that makes you happy, satisfied, even joyous. That has more of an effect on your economic well-being than any other single factor."
-Paul Hawken

"The purpose of our lives is to be happy."
-Dalai Lama

"There is no way to happiness; happiness is the way."
-Buddha

Happiness Resources

www.thewaytohappiness.org

www.happinessinfusion.com

www.aarp.org/health-tips

www.improvingyourworld.com

www.motivationandhappiness.com

www.thehappyguy.com

www.psychologytoday.com/basics/happiness

www.happinesspodcast.org

http://happiness-project.com

http://sohp.com

www.ingramcontent.com/pod-product-compliance
Lightning Source LLC
Chambersburg PA
CBHW070820290526
45795CB00002B/786